All you need to know...

About diabetes

Garth Howell

Please note that much of this publication is based on personal experience and research. Although the author and publisher have made every reasonable attempt to achieve complete accuracy of the content in this Guide, they assume no responsibility for errors or omissions. Also, you should use this information as you see fit, and at your own risk. If you are in doubt the please seek the advice of a medical professional. Your particular situation may not be exactly suited to the examples illustrated here; in fact, it's likely that they won't be the same, and you should adjust your use of the information and recommendations accordingly

Other works by Garth Howell

Sleep apnea, symptoms, diagnosis and treatment

Available from Createspace

https://www.createspace.com/3959267

What is type 2 diabetes?

The subject of diabetes to many people is very confusing. The first thing we must consider is, is what diabetes is and what constitutes a diagnosis. There are many myths associated with the condition and the aim of this publication is explain diabetes and to expose the the many myths surrounding the condition.

Diabetes is a condition in which there is an excess of glucose (a type of sugar) in the blood.

There are 2 types of diabetes 1 & 2, this book is about type 2 diabetes.

The amount of glucose in the blood is controlled by insulin which is a hormone produced by the pancreas and with type 2 diabetes the pancreas produces insulin but unfortunately the body is not able to use it correctly and the condition is known as insulin resistance.

Diabetes can progress if the pancreas starts to produce less insulin thus it is a condition that needs to be carefully monitored and controlled.

The problem is that if too much glucose is present in the blood, the blood will become thicker and sticky, as if you dissolve sugar in water. This can have an effect on the body, which if unchecked can have serious consequences. It is therefore very important to ensure that the amount of glucose present in the blood is kept under control. Once you have been diagnosed as having diabetes it will not go away but keeping it under control will enable you to limit the consequences.

The Glucose story

To understand diabetes it is necessary to understand glucose, which is produced when the food we have eaten is broken down in the stomach.

The glucose then travels around the body in the bloodstream.

Some glucose is stored in the liver and is gradually released during the day and night.

Insulin, produced by the pancreas acts like a key and opens doors so that glucose is able to get into cells to produce energy.

Diabetes is caused when the glucose is not broken down into energy either by insufficient insulin or insulin resistance. To control diabetes it is therefore necessary to both monitor and control the amount of glucose in the bloodstream.

Symptoms of diabetes

The symptoms of diabetes can be can be varied and developing all or just one of the symptoms listed below can be can be a sign that your glucose levels are high.

Here is a list of some of the more common symptoms which can be caused if glucose levels are elevated

- Feeling thirsty

- Repeated infections

- Tiredness

- Blurred vision

- For men - having difficulty getting erections

- Needing to pass urine more than normal or in the night

- Itching of the skin, especially the genital area.

- Slow healing of cuts and wounds

- Abnormal weight loss.

With type 2 diabetes the symptoms may come on very slowly you may not even notice them, it can be that they are picked up when you have a routine medical check. If you notice any of these, and are concerned I would recommend that you contact your doctor and have your glucose levels checked.

In some cases a person may be diagnosed as diabetic without any of these symptoms and this may well mean that they are in the very early stages of the condition.

Diagnosis of diabetes

The diagnosis of diabetes will be made by your Doctor who after looking at your medical history will want to make a series of checks.

Firstly a urine sample will be taken and the urine tested for glucose. It is likely that a blood sample will be taken after you have fasted, normally this is done first thing in the morning. A glycosylated haemoglobin test (HbA1C) may also be carried out. HbA1C is a protein that can appear in the blood if glucose levels have been high for a prolonged time.

A glucose tolerance test may also be carried out if your fasting blood test is borderline. Again this is a test which is carried out after fasting overnight. A blood sample is taken followed by you drinking a sugary glucose drink. You then wait for 2 hours when a further blood test is taken. The two blood sample test how your blood sugar varies over time.

Many people are quite understandably very frightened and upset when they discover they have type 2 diabetes. It is true that left unchecked diabetes can have serious consequences but there are ways in which the condition can be managed and enable the sufferer to live without serious inconvenience.

Management and treatment of diabetes

The nature of diabetes means that the management and treatment of diabetes can be very different from person to person as can the effects. There are however some fairly simple changes to your life that you can make which may well enable you to control your blood sugar levels.

Ensure that you eat a balanced diet and eat regularly. Include all the food types in your diet but in moderation. If you are overweight, your insulin resistance can be improved by shedding a few pounds.

Increase your physical activity to help control your blood sugar levels. A good target is to do at least 150 minutes of exercise a week carried out in a minimum of 10 minute sessions. To obtain the most benefit from exercise you need to carry out a minimum of 10 minutes fairly brisk exercises and several short sessions is better for you than taking an hour a couple of times a week.

Manage your alcohol consumption to within reasonable limits.

It is also worth stopping smoking to avoid damage to the circulatory system.

If your levels of glucose won't respond to the above then there are various medications available. Metformin can be prescribed to improve insulin resistance. There are medications known as glitazones which can help make the body more sensitive to insulin and a group of drugs called sulphonylureas which help the pancreas to produce insulin.

Over time you may need injections of drugs such as exenatide or liraglutide which help the body produce insulin and also help with weight loss.

It may be however that changes in your lifestyle and the taking of prescribed drugs is still not sufficient to control your diabetes and you may require insulin in either tablet or injection form. There are different types of insulin that work at different rates and your Doctor will advise which is the best for you.

If you do take insulin it will be necessary to monitor your blood glucose levels at home with a test kit. This involves a small prick of the finger to obtain a drop of blood which goes onto a test strip. A meter will tell you what your levels are. You will be shown how to use this by either your doctor or a diabetes nurse.

Risks and complications of diabetes

You often hear people say that they have diabetes but it is only mild. Unfortunately there is no such thing as mild diabetes as such. If you have diabetes that is not under control you are exposing yourself to severe risks.

Risks associated with diabetes

Diabetes if unchecked can causes damage to the blood vessels both large and small and nerves. The high blood sugar level as previously described can make the blood sticky and glucose can stick to the sides of blood vessels causing a furring up and a hardening. This can causes the small blood vessels to narrow and to clog up and this can cause problems to to various parts of the body.

- Eyes – Retina damage can be caused which can cause blindness.

- Kidneys – Damage to the kidneys can cause failure

- Nerve damage – called diabetic neuropathy can cause foot sores and ulcers which can in turn create the need for leg and foot amputations.

- Damage to the nerves in the autonomic nervous system which can result in heart problems and blood pressure problems when changing posture and also chronic diarrhoea caused by the paralysis of the stomach.

- Blood clots can be caused leading to strokes and heart attacks or lack of blood to the legs and feet.

- Diabetes can make you more likely to suffer from raised blood pressure, raised cholesterol and raised triglycerides.

- If the blood sugar gets very high the body will try to get rid of it through the urine. In doing so urine production may be increased which in turn can cause dehydration which can lead to seizure's, coma's or even death. This is known as hyperosmolar hyperglycemic nonketotic syndrome.

Take control of the situation

If you have been diagnosed as being diabetic it is necessary to take some control over your life. There are several things that you can do to now that you know the risk factors and complications associated with the condition.

Do not think you are alone. There are many people suffering from type 2 diabetes who manage to lead good quality lives and there is support out there. Your healthcare providers in the form of your Doctor or Diabetic nurse are there to help you and there are also many support groups and forums where you can go to for either help or advice.

You may decided that now is the time to make a few changes which will not only benefit your health but also help control your diabetes.

1 Reduce Blood Glucose

Try to control and reduce your blood glucose by eating less and eating smaller portions, particularly of starchy carbohydrate and eat foods that break down into glucose more slowly. These are the low Glycemic Index foods and it is well worth becoming familiar with what these are. Be careful about the amount of fats you consume and helps to lose weight and reduce the circumference of your waist. Taking more exercise will also help to reduce blood glucose levels

2. Stop Smoking

If you are a smoker try to stop and if that proves difficult to do alone then seek help and try one or more of the many products there are to assist in the reducing of craving of nicotine.

3. Reduce Blood Pressure

If your blood pressure is outside the normal range of 120/80 then it is important to try to get it to within the norm. On diagnosis your medical practitioner should have checked your blood pressure and given you advice. There are however things that you can do to help the situation.

If your Doctor has prescribed medication then be sure to take it.

4. Lowering Cholesterol

It is important to maintain your cholesterol levels to within the recommended range which is below 200mg/dl in US measurement or below 5.20mml/ltre.

It is likely that your medical practitioner will have checked this on diagnosis and if high will have prescribed medication, normally statins. You can help control cholesterol by eating less fat and more fruit and vegetables and being more active.

5. Lose weight

If overweight then it is advisable to try to reduce weight and reduce the waist measurement. Eating smaller portions may help, as will eating less fat and drinking less alcohol. Again, becoming physically active too will help you to burn calories.

6. Reduce Depression

Being depressed and suffering from stress will not help your diabetes. If you are depressed then it is advisable that you seek some help.

7. Look after circulation and blood vessels

We have looked at the effect of raised blood glucose levels on blood vessels and it is worth keeping them in the best condition that you can. Certainly dealing with topics 1-6 will help and it is advisable to eat 2-4 portions of oily fish per week and some suggest taking an aspirin a day may help also but seek advice before doing so as aspirin can have unpleasant side effects when taken regularly.

The Diabetic annual review

If you have been diagnosed with type 2 diabetes you should be offered an annual review where your condition will be monitored. It will also be used to check blood glucose levels, cholesterol levels and measure blood pressure. If you are newly diagnosed or there could be possible complications then your condition will be reviewed more often.

At the review the medical practitioner will carry out the following:-

Measure your height and weight

Check your blood pressure

Review blood glucose control

Review HbA1c and cholesterol levels

The kidneys will also be checked by measuring the amount of protein in the urine.

Foot check

Best to ensure they are clean before the appointment. Your feet will be checked for general condition particularly if there are any ulcers. Any blisters or ingrowing toenails will also be noted. You will also be asked if you have any sensory nerve loss and a small microfilament will be brushed across the surface of the skin and you will be asked if you have any sensation.

The capillary return will also be checked by pressing on the nail beds for 5 seconds. The nail should turn from pink to red in less than 3 seconds.

The palpation of the foot arteries, the posterior libial and the dorsalis pedis and whether the feet are warm or not.

If it looks as if there may be foot problems then more tests will be carried in order that any damage can be assessed.

You should also be offered an eye test annually to check for macular degeneration. Here drops are put into the eye to widen the pupil and the retina examined. Photographs are usually also taken for reference purposes so that any deterioration may be noticed over time. The drops can cause blurred vision and you must not drive for 4-6 hours after the test. It is a good idea to ask someone to accompany you when you have this test.

If you do suffer from diabetes then do not miss the annual checks and reviews, they may be your life saver.

The myths associated with diabetes

Having taken a look at diabetes I think that we should knock down a few of the myths that are often associated with the condition.

1) Eating too much sugar causes diabetes

The first myth is that eating too much sugar causes diabetes. This is simply not true. When you have diabetes the production of insulin and the way that your body uses changes. When you have diabetes the body still produces insulin but either it is not enough or it is not used effectively enough. As already explained too much glucose in the blood causes damage to the body organs over time and as the glucose stays in the blood you don't receive the energy that you require. Carbohydrates in food is where you get your energy from and carbohydrates get broken down into glucose. It is therefore better to eat carbohydrates that break down slowly over a period of time such as wholemeal products and vegetables and avoid eating processed food where possible. I have dealt with Glycemic Index for foods earlier in this book. There is no need to give up eating the food you like just because you have diabetes. Just fit it in as part of an overall plan.

2) If you are overweight you will eventually contract diabetes

This is a common myth and the truth is that many overweight people never contract diabetes. In reality being overweight can and does cause health problems such as high blood pressure, heart disease strokes and respiratory problems to name a few. It will also make you more liable to become diabetic. It is a fact that many overweight people become diabetic because their insulin production is unable to cope. If weight is lost then things revert back to normal This however does not mean that you are not diabetic as one you are diabetic then you stay diabetic but being overweight will not cause diabetes in itself.

3) Type 2 is a mild form of diabetes

Diabetes is a serious condition and should be treated seriously. The major differences are that in type 1 diabetes the body produces no diabetes and insulin needs to be injected to provided the body with it. In type 2 the body produces insulin but not enough and the cells do not use it as effectively as they should. Type 1 is sometimes referred to as juvenile diabetes as it is normally diagnosed at an early age whereas type 2 is known as late onset and is a progressive disease where the body will change over a period of time although lifestyle changes can keep the condition under control.

4) Diabetics should eat diabetic food

I'm afraid diabetic food is just a ploy by the marketing men. Most of the foods that are labelled diabetic foods do not taste as good, because instead of adding any sugar sweetening has been added instead or reduced sugar and the price has been increased. Enjoy your food in moderation and eat a controlled diet.

5) People with diabetes will eventually go blind

This is a myth that terrifies most people and it is certainly true that if your glucose levels are not controlled you may cause eye damage. If you have regular eye checks and live a healthy life this should keep the serious effects of diabetes away.

6) If you have diabetes you must soak your feet daily As already explained it is important to look after your feet and regularly check for cuts and sores and react if breaks in the skin are not healing quickly. You do not however have to soak

you feet on a daily basis, in fact soaking your feet may cause the skin to be more prone to damage.

7) Insulin can cause men to become impotent

Insulin will never cause erectile dis-function, The cause of impotence in men is caused by nerve damage due to constant high glucose levels.

8) You can catch diabetes from another person

Diabetes is not a contagious condition. You cannot catch it from another person. You may however have a similar body type to a relative making you predisposed to becoming diabetic yourself.

9) Diabetics are more likely to catch colds or flu

There is no reason to believe that diabetics are more likely to catch colds or flu. It is however possible that if you do it could cause your blood glucose levels to rise quite dramatically. If you do catch a cold then just do a bit of extra monitoring.

10) You can eat as much fruit as you like.

Fruits contain vitamins and fibre. Unfortunately they also contain a lot of fructose which is a natural sugar. If you like eating fruit spread it out over they day to avoid you getting glucose level spikes.

11) Diabetes can be cured through diet

This statement is totally false. There is no "cure" for diabetes all you can do is to keep it under control. And in any cases this can be done by diet. People have been diagnosed as diabetic, lost some weight and suddenly they find that the symptoms of diabetes have disappeared. What has happened here is that they have demonstrated themselves to be insulin resistant in some way due to being over weight. They are still diabetic and need to keep watching their glucose levels and maintaining a healthy lifestyle.

12) You can be borderline diabetic

A most definite no here. You are either diabetic or you are not.

13) Diabetics can no longer play sport

That statement is totally untrue. The opposite is in fact the case as healthy activity is to be encouraged. If you engaged in physical activity you are burning off calories and also excess glucose present in the blood. It is important to monitor your exercise as if you have not been active for a long time too much activity all at once could be damaging. Keep active.

14) It is not safe to drive if you are diabetic

If you diabetes is under control and you are not suffering from sight problems, dizzy spells or hypos then you are as safe to drive as anyone else. It really is about common sense. No one should drive if they feel unwell.

15) Diabetics should not eat certain fruits

Some fruits are higher in sugar than others such as melons, grapes and pineapple. This doesn't however mean that you cant eat them. Just be sensible and eat them as part of a controlled diet.

16) Diabetics should not cut their own toe nails

They are your feet and possibly you are the best person to deal with them so there is no truth in that statement. Do however be careful and try not to break the skin in the process.

17) You should not eat sugary products

This is a common myth as people associate diabetes with sugar. It has already been mentioned that carbohydrates turn into glucose which the body then uses as fuel to regenerate the cells. The link to sugar comes from the the fact that the urine from some diabetics has a sweet smell which gave the condition the term sugar diabetes. Eating too much sugar won't give you diabetes per se.

18) You should never eat chocolate

This myth is linked to the one above. Nobody whether they are diabetic or not should be consuming large amounts of chocolate as there are a large number of calories in each bar. In moderation however to eat some chocolate will do you no harm as long as it fits into the overall diet plan. Don't think that diabetic chocolate is better for you because it is more expensive and doesn't taste as good. Have a little of the real thing.

If you have to go onto insulin you are not looking after yourself properly

Type 2 diabetes will progress as you get older. You may be able to keep your condition under control but inevitably as time goes on your condition will change and you may have to go onto insulin. This is no reflection on you , its just that the body is no longer producing adequate insulin to keep your blood glucose levels in the safety zone.

19) You should never take aspirin if diabetic

There is research being carried out as whether aspirin is safe for diabetics but at the time of rating it is considered safe to take aspirin if you are diabetic. I would however be cautious and check with your doctor before doing so. He will be able to give you the up to date advice.

20) If you are diagnosed as diabetic then you are doomed

Many people think that if they are diagnosed as being diabetic then they are doomed. The most important thing is to recognise you have this condition which has the potential to do serious damage and react accordingly by following a sensible eating plan, exercise and generally live a healthy life. That should keep the effects of diabetes at bay and enable you to lead a fulfilled life.

Moving Forward

So you have been diagnosed as having type 2 diabetes, it may well have been a bit of a shock and if you are like the majority of people you will have experienced the following symptoms.

Relief

This is quite natural because now you actually know why you have not been feeling quite right. You have an answer and you can now move on to putting in a plan to deal with the problem

Denial

You probably have a niggling feeling that just maybe you haven't got diabetes. You may well have always been fit, nor overweight. You don't like sugary foods. Here are the diabetes myths coming into play. If you go through denial it is usually a link to having false knowledge of the condition.

Depression

I think many people go through this in some way. It is important to understand and accept that you have to spend the rest of your life with this condition and things will never quite be the same again. If you are depressed about it don't bear it alone but seek help for it is only when you can get through the depression you will arrive at the acceptance stage when you can go on lead a fulfilled life again.

Acceptance

Once you have accepted that you suffer from diabetes you can move forward and take control of your life again and your management of the condition will be so much more effective.

Diabetes medication

If, on your review it is discovered that your blood sugar levels are not under control by controlling your diet and taking exercise iit is likely that you will require medication to assist. Over time it is likely that your diabetes will worsen and lifestyle modifcation is no longer enough. Initially any medication is likely to be in the form of a tablet or combination of more than one type of tablet. It may at some stage also involve you having to inject insulin.

There are several different types of medication but initially you are likely to be precribed Metaformin.

Metaformin

Metaformin is usually the first medication to be prescribed to treat diabetes and comes in the form of a tablet. Metaformin works by reducing the amount of glucose released into the bloodstream by the liver.

There may be side effects from using Metaformin although they are usually mild and take the form of nausea and diarrhoea but it will not cause weight gain. If you already have kidney damage however you may not be prescribed with Metaformin.

Sulphonylureas

If you are unable to take Metaformin or your wight is not a problem you may be prescribed Sulphonylureas. You may also be prescribed one of the Sulhonylureas along with Metaformin if the the Metaformin does not work on its ownin the control of your blood sugar.

Sulphonylureas work by increasing the amount of insulin in your body and like may drugs can have side effects. These can include nausea. Diarrhoea and weight gain. Examples of Sulphonylureas are glibenclamide, gliciazide and glipizide.

Glitazones (thiazolidinediones, TZDs)

This group of drugs work by making the body cells more sensitive to insulin thus more glucose is taken from the blood. They are usually used in conjunction with other medications.

Glitazones can cause swollen ankles and weight gain and should not be taken if you have heart failure or your bones are likely to fracture.

Gliptins, GLP-1 Agonsists, Acarbose are other medications that may be prescribed to control diabetes and there are some others. It is really important that you work with your medical advisers to find the the best medication for you.

Insulin Treatment

It is possible that glucose controlling medications are not enough to control your diabetes and if this is the case then you you may take it alongside exisiting medication. There are different preparations of insulin as some are long acting and last the whole day and some just act for a few hours. Treatment can be made up of a combination of the different insulin preparations.

In most cases insulin is injected as if it were taken orally it would need to, like food be broken down in the stomach and it would not be able to enter the blood stream.

Insuli injections can be made either using a syringe or an injection (insulin) pen. Injections are usually required either 2 or 4 times per day.

Instruction on injecting will be given by your medical practitioner.

Other Treatment

Your risk of heart disease, stroke and kdney disease is increased if you are diabetic and it is very likely that along with your diabetes monitoring your blood pressure and cholesterol levels will also be monitored.

If your blood pressure is above the range 120/80 you will probably be prescribed medication to control it.

You may also be precribed a statin to keep your cholesterol under control or if your cholesterol is high to reduce it.

Low dose aspirin to help to avoid a stroke.

Your kidney function is also likely to be monitored by testing for albumin which is a protein in the urine. If you have early signs of diabetic kidney disease you may be prescribed and ACE inhihibitor such as lisinopril. Early detection does mean you have a much greater chance of any kidney disease being reversed.

Self Help

As well as taking all the usual measures to either try to avoid or control diabetes if you are diagnosed there are other measures that you can take which may help.

The usual measures which have already been dealt with are to, manage your weight, eat a diet low in sugars and carbohydrates and eat plenty of lean protein, vegetables and wholegrains.

There are however a few other measures that are believed to help.

Cinnamon

Research has been carried out on the effect of cinnamon on humans. 60 people too either 1,3 or 6 gms of cinnamon per day in the form of a tablet. (1 tablet=approx 1tsp ground cinnamon). After 40 days it was discovered that the fasting blood glucose level was reduced from by 18 to 29%, triglycerides by 23 to 30%, bad cholesterol (LDL) by 7 to 27% and total cholesterol by 12 to 26%. This applied to all 3 amounts of cinnamon. (Source: Diabetes care 2003).

Other tests have been carried out. One of these was a Swedish study where people were given rice pudding either with or without cinnamon added. It was shown that the after eating rise in blood sugar was lowered in those who had the cinnamon compared to those who did not. (Source: American Journal of Clinical Nutrition). The sample was however very small at just 14 people.

It may therefore be worthwhile to add a little cinnamon to your diet, it's a delicious spice. Be warned however that high consumption can cause liver damage, and in some forms it has blood thinning properties.

Chromium

Chromium supplement appears to be quite useful in helping to control your glucose levels. There is a molecule in the body called glucose-tolerance factor and chromium is a component of it. It is known to enhance the action of insulin in lowering blood sugar.

Animal studies have shown that a chromium deficient diet results in high blood sugar levels.

Sources of Chromium in food are mushrooms, brewers yeast, and eggs. It may be worth taking a supplement in the form of tablets available fro health food stores. Normally the tablets are 200 micrograms and the normal dose is one daily. The better absorbed forms are Chromium aspartate, chromium picolinate, and chromium polynicotinate.

Some believe that to be really effective 200 micrograms is not enough and needs to be around 500. I would advise the reader to carry out their own research and seek advice regarding this.

Summary

To sum up, diabetes is a dangerous condition. It may be that you are diabetic already or perhaps your lifestyle means that you are running the risk of becoming a diabetic. You may be young or old. You can however do your health and wellbeing a great service by leading a healthy lifestyle.

Take control of your own health and wellbeing, there is a lot you can do to help yourself.

The book has demonstrated that in most cases extreme measures are not required. What will help however is to apply common sense, control carbohydates, sugars and fat intake and lead an active life. If you do this you will help your life chances.

If you are diagnosed as diabetic it does not mean the end. You should be able to lead a full and active life.

Thank you for reading.